THE REALIST'S GUIDE TO SUGAR-FREE

HOW TO QUIT SUGAR AND STAY SANE IN THE REAL WORLD

SHERRI NICHOLDS

First published 2016

ISBN-13: 9781520534138

DISCLAIMER

I am not a doctor. I am not a nutritionist. This book is not intended as a substitute for the medical advice of physicians. You should consult a physician before embarking on any kind of diet or exercise programme, especially if you have any known medical conditions.

I have also written this without any references to food allergies or intolerances. These are very real problems for many people, so please do not deviate from any traditional approaches you may have for dealing with these as a result of this book without consulting your medical professional.

Finally, the opinions contained herein are mine, and do not represent those of any company or client I work for.

CONTENTS

INTRODUCTION

I've been on the sugar-free journey for about a year. It
has been an experience with many ups and downs, but
along the way I have become consumed by the idea of
getting sugar out of my life.

As the world is slowly becoming more aware of the
impact of sugar on our waistlines and then our
healthcare systems, more and more people are
considering the possibility of going sugar-free. Some
doctors are beginning to advise people with a whole
spectrum of conditions to do so. So I decided to write
this book to give people a helping hand. Why? Because
the one thing I have learned along the way is this:
quitting sugar is *hard*.

The Realist's Guide To Sugar-Free isn't a cookbook, it's not
a science book and it's certainly not a fad diet book. I
am a sample size of one, unless you include some of my
friends who have also tried it and fallen off the wagon
many times along the way. I've failed to maintain a
sugar-free life *twice* in the space of that year, so I can tell

you up front - holidays are going to be tough.

There's already a booming market in books about cutting sugar from your diet, so why did I feel the need to write another one to add to the list? Especially one that doesn't even fall into the categories I've described above? Quite simply, although there were many very good titles to choose from, I didn't feel most of them captured the everyday reality for a lot of people living a normal 'western' lifestyle. Although I'm writing this from England, the way of eating is broadly the same as across the USA, Australia and sadly, an increasing number of European countries as well. Those countries that have traditionally been lauded as healthy diet countries are now falling into our bad ways and as a result, the obesity rates are going through the roof. So this book has been written with the reality of big food companies - and not enough time each day - in mind. My goal is to give you the information you need to be able to give up sugar for good. It is an honest approach. It will be realistic, sharing both the good and bad sides to this new journey you're about to embark upon. There are no shortcuts to be found here. Only helpful advice to get you started and keep you going.

A lot of countries provide a respectable level of

healthcare coverage, such as the NHS does in the UK. Sadly, the financial burden of running this has reached almost breaking point. Some would say it has already broken and we just haven't faced up to the fact yet. I hope private healthcare as the only option never happens here, but if it does, then let me tell you this: you don't want to be paying a fortune to cover you for sugar related illnesses such as heart disease and diabetes. Do the work now, just in case. That's all I'm saying.

If you're like me, you might even question if you need to go sugar-free after all. I have always seen myself as a 'savoury' person. The vast majority of the time, I gravitate towards crisps and cheese rather than chocolate and cake. For years, I also thought I was a healthy eater. But when I started looking closely, all those sauces and dressings for my burgers and salads contained mind-boggling amounts of sugar. Worse, all of those low cal, low fat foods contained epic amounts of the white stuff (more on that later).

So the only people who won't need this book are the following:

People who don't eat any processed foods

That's it. List of one. It doesn't matter if you are a sweet person or a savoury person, healthy or unhealthy. If you are buying pretty much anything that comes in a packet, jar, tin or bottle, someone will have helpfully already added that sugar in for you and unless you take a really close look at the label, then you won't have a clue.

The odds are stacked against you right from the start my friend. Your body will rebel against you. Food companies will push ever tastier treats onto the market that you won't be able to have. Going to a restaurant will often mean a menu choice of one. Your friends will recoil in horror at the prospect of knowing someone who no longer eats chocolate and is refusing a slice of cake. It will be tough, but I want to show you how to face those odds and still win. That's why I didn't put a picture on the cover of a skinny model - with impossibly glowing skin - laughing at a plate of food that takes four hours to prepare and contains ingredients no one knows how to pronounce.

This book is to guide you through the lessons I've learnt the hard way, so that you don't have to make the same mistakes. It's realistic. It's honest. Being unhealthy is far easier, which is why so many of us are and continue to remain that way.

But if you think you're tough enough, read on...

CHAPTER ONE: WHY GO SUGAR-FREE?

I'm not a doctor, nutritionist or biochemist. This is not a science book. I've written this book on the premise that you've already pretty much decided to give living sugar-free a go and you just need a sensible place to start. Or perhaps you've become curious and need more information without having to get a biochemistry degree and have a Michelin starred chef to hand. But if you've just seen that some celebrities are doing it and you want to see what all the fuss is about, then let me give you a very quick overview.

In terms of our body, it is fructose that does the most damage. Fructose is a component element of sugar, so this is never listed on any nutrition labels. Given that it makes up half of the white stuff that we think of as sugar, it is more realistic in daily life to attempt to go 'sugar-free' rather than 'fructose-free'. Despite the origins of the name fructose, this book is not going to demonise whole fruit either. For the purpose of actually being able to live in the real world, I'm not going to expect you to eat no sugar at all, ever again. Sugar-free will be 10g of sugar or less per day. That's still not a small amount, but you'll get up to it very, very quickly. The composition of your 10g of sugar will vary the impacts, too, but for now, having this as a generic lifestyle goal will put you miles ahead of the competition anyway.

This chapter poses the simple question, why go sugar-free? The reason I've pointed out straight away that I'm not a doctor or any kind of expert in this area in some ways is irrelevant, because even the people with impressive degrees don't yet one hundred per cent agree on the best approach to take. As a non-scientist, I always thought the beauty of the subject was that it was black or white. Correct or incorrect. Not like literature, where if you could waffle on convincingly about the symbolic meaning of a rose, then you'd probably get some points in an exam. Science was meant to be the serious stuff, with clear lines.

Not so.

Firstly, science is expensive. So you'll find that most science requires significant funding. Funding that often comes, either directly or indirectly, from people with an agenda. In this case, food manufacturers. It's surprising how many executives of food companies sit on health advisory boards and no one has batted an eyelid at the potential conflict of interest. This is one of the many reasons the modern world has been so slow to wake up to the dangers of our sugar consumption.

You don't know what they don't want you to know.

There are two myths, as I see them, about our modern diet and everything we've been told about nutrition that we need to break. We need to bring them out into the open and expose them. They are so engrained into the way we think about our food, it has become nothing more than a habit to look at eating this way, especially when we're trying to lose weight. In fact, losing weight is the only reason many people think about food choices at all. This chapter shows the impact of sugar on health, not clothes size. Sugar can be quietly killing you with your normal BMI and skinny jeans too.

Myth one - a calorie is a calorie.

That is the first thing you'll have to change your way of thinking about. It's harder than it seems; after all, the answer to losing weight in our lifetime has always been simple: eat a calorie controlled diet and exercise. Calories are listed everywhere. They are the key labelling information on any food product, right there at the top. Daily recommended amounts for men and women, in curiously convenient round numbers.

Don't get me wrong. Chances are if you eat 10,000 calories a day, whilst sitting around doing nothing, I completely get that you're going to start piling on the pounds. I'm not disputing that at all. But what science is increasingly showing is that a calorie is a calorie, *inside the lab*. Inside the human body, it's a completely different thing altogether.

This is where I run into a difficulty. I need to go into enough detail to be convincing, but not so technical that you get bored and start skipping along to the next chapter. Trust me, I've read those books too. But if you don't know about this already, understanding why sugar behaves differently is the key to getting the motivation to give it up.

I'm assuming that some of you reading this have children, and virtually all of you reading this used to be children. If you don't fall into either bracket, then get in touch and I can make millions writing about you instead. So, on that assumption, I'm going to make it all clear using... Lego.

Yes, that's right. Who doesn't understand Lego?

Food gets broken down by our bodies to produce energy. We know that much, we all sat through that lesson at school. But it's the breaking down bit that's interesting.

No matter what you are eating, whether you're chilling out on a Saturday night in junk food heaven or being virtuous on Monday lunchtime with a quinoa and beetroot salad, once the food is broken down, it can only fall into one of three types that the body uses for energy: protein, fat or carbohydrate. We're not bothered about protein and fat right now (although you'll see how they increase in importance later). Sugars are part of the carbohydrate group, so for what we need to know, this is where we start looking. Carbohydrates themselves can be broken down into three main simple types of sugars:

Glucose - let's call this a green brick

Galactose - this is found in dairy products like milk, so let's call this one a yellow brick

Fructose - this is the little guy we need to be concerned about, so he gets to be nature's warning colour - red

The reason a calorie is not a calorie is because of the way the body handles these little bricks of energy.

Glucose is the main source our body uses. We need it to get us through our everyday lives, our brains use it in huge quantities (relatively speaking) to think, and it's a handy thing that our body likes to store so if we get up and can't find anything to eat when we're out hunting and gathering, we don't just drop down dead on the spot. Glucose is the main man according to our bodies. It sees those little bricks of green Lego and sends them off to the various sites where they can be used. We Lego-fort our brains and muscles in green and our body is happy with that. It knows green. It understands green. It sees the value of green and knows how many bricks you've eaten. Okay, the analogy had to break down somewhere. Do not consume children's toys as part of the sugar-free diet.

Galactose, our lovely yellow Lego, works in a similar way. When people are intolerant to dairy, this yellow brick is what they don't like. They can't process it and end up passing it out of the system. (There's a shitting bricks part of this analogy too then apparently). For those of us who don't have any intolerances, a yellow brick is like a green brick to our body. We can break it down and happily use it to supplement those green bricks as we build our fort. Our muscles and brain do all the heavy lifting to stack it up and knock it down.

So why is fructose different?

When those red bricks go into our body, our brain and muscles don't play with them in the same way. Our appetite hormones are blissfully unaware of them. Only our liver can really play with the red bricks and when you start eating a lot of them, then that suddenly becomes a lot of pressure to put on one organ in your body. Besides, your liver only needs two or three bricks to be happy and instead we eat like we've got a bumper box of Lego for our birthday and it contained mainly red bricks. It needs to do something with them and it can't use them all. The liver is too small a place to build a really big fort. So it's working away trying to get rid of them and while this is going on, because we don't see fructose with our appetite hormones, the rest of our body is blissfully unaware of what is going on (more on why that's a problem in chapter two).

This is the calorie you don't see. This is the calorie that is not a calorie, because you don't use it like the other bricks. This is the calorie that, unless you are in complete deficit of green and yellow bricks, your body has to dump somewhere. So it does.

As fat.

Myth two - fat makes you fat.

Hello myth number two. Good to see you. This is the one that, after growing up in a 'low fat diet' culture, I still really struggle to break away from on a daily basis. It is embedded deep into my thinking. Sadly, it is largely based on the advice of a study that has recently been shown to have a few errors that even I know shouldn't be made when doing science. You know, like discounting the things that don't go along with your hypothesis and pretending they aren't there. Plus being paid by those very people who have an interest in getting you to eat their tasty, tasty sweet food.

It's been presented to us very simplistically, almost as though food doesn't go through any kind of digestion process. We happily imagine eating fat and our bodies gleefully throwing it straight onto our thighs. Or belly. Pick your own body part of engrained societal pressured self-loathing.

Again, I'm not saying that you can eat as much excess fat as you like and it doesn't matter. Not at all. You eat more than your body can use or get rid of, it's going to put it somewhere. But the simple equation that we've been presented of lots of fat in diet equals fat person is horribly simplistic. Fat should be, and always was until the last century, a significant part of our diet. Other carnivorous and omnivorous mammals do not avoid fat.

So what role does sugar play then, if being healthy is not about calories and fat?

Your liver, the only place in the body that can play with the red bricks, does what it can. It takes that fructose, uses what it needs and then gets to work processing it off along the way. The output? Fatty acids mainly. Some of these your body can use. Your body is the product of millennia of evolution, so it does what it can, with what it has, in the most efficient way. But it doesn't need a lot and all that fatty acid in your bloodstream has to get dumped somewhere, and that somewhere is the body part you identified earlier, along with sticking to a couple of other places, like your arteries, slowly clogging them up. Or your liver, leaving fatty deposits and scarring until it can no longer work as efficiently at keeping your body running smoothly and getting rid of poisons.

Grossed out yet?

Research is only really just beginning to emerge about this. For decades, the 'low fat, more exercise' approach was recited so much, everyone just took it for granted, including scientists and nutritionists. Many of them still do. Did you know that most GPs, for example, will have had perhaps a single lecture on diet and nutrition as part of qualifying? Strange that something so integral to human health factors so low on the learning scale. Now, based on these long held beliefs, in the western world, more people are eating 'low fat' foods, more people are going to the gym to frantically burn off calories more than ever before, yet obesity is still catastrophically on the rise. Not just in adults, but in kids too. For most adults I know, it is a conscious effort not to get fat just from existing, even if they spend all day running around after their children and (increasingly) aging parents and living the opposite of the sedentary life we've all been accused of.

The thing that's changed the most? Sugar consumption.

Over the past two hundred years, the average American went from consuming approximately 6lbs of sugar per year, up to approximately 107lbs per year by the time we partied like it was 1999. That is a significant dietary change.

Now that scientists are starting to overcome the stigma of breaking away from the culture of low fat, research is beginning into the links between sugar consumption and diseases that are on the rise. Fledgling studies are beginning to look towards proving that sugar has an impact on not only metabolic syndrome and diabetes, but also:

- Heart diseases
- Fatty liver diseases
- Pancreatic diseases
- Several types of cancer
- Female fertility problems
- Autism
- Alzheimer's disease

These are all chronic conditions that have been dramatically on the rise. What if all of these could be reduced or avoided by the removal of sugar? It would be a scenario with massive implications for our lives, our healthcare systems and most importantly, the next generations.

On a side note, one of the reasons why I wanted to write this book, why I felt compelled to do whatever little bit I can, even if I only help one person to break the sugar addiction, was the discovery that sugar is added to baby formula. Why? Babies don't have a sweet tooth. They don't have any teeth at all for that matter. Yet we are literally setting up generation after generation to crave sweet food. Hardwiring the brain from birth to be consumers of a product that doesn't happen in food naturally (obviously with the exception of fruit, which has fibre built into the package to slow down that hit on your liver). This means that like all addicts, we're happy to purchase our fix.

These companies aren't billion dollar corporations because they are stupid. They are very, very smart. And they've been pulling the wool over our eyes for years.

As I promised (even though it might not feel like it) this is a *very* high level overview, for those who just wanted a bit more background. Not a scientific argument, with points for and against the theory. It'll actually feel normal to challenge it as you read it, because the myths are part of our psyche and way of life. If you want to go into more depth, but without going into the kind of science that is meaningless to all but the brainiest on the planet, then I can highly recommend *Sweet Poison* by David Gillespie. It's a fantastic book for those wanting to understand and maintain a real sense of why they need to keep moving on this journey.

If you're thinking to yourself that all of this makes sense, so why not just cut out the sugar, then it's time to move to the next kick in the pants. Not only is sugar bad for you, there are a whole host of reasons why it's so hard to stop eating it. Understanding the damage it is doing to your system is one thing, beating the hold it has over you is another. This is why I've written the *realist's* guide, remember? Because as you're about to find out, you don't just stop eating sugar. It's far too clever to let you do that.

CHAPTER TWO: I CAN QUIT ANY TIME

According to some reports, sugar is as addictive as crack cocaine. Just take a moment to think about that.

Crack cocaine.

Now, I don't know any crack addicts, but they don't exactly have a reputation for being able to stop at any time. Also, you have to make a conscious effort to try crack in the first place before you get addicted to it.

Not so with sugar. Sugar is everywhere. You don't need to do a dodgy deal with someone to procure a bit, furtively looking over your shoulder as someone discretely hands over a bag of Tate & Lyle. The most drama involved in getting your sugar fix in the morning is pouring a bowl of cereal. There's no conscious thought involved. We feed our addiction every single day without realising it.

As yet, there's no twelve step programme for breaking the sugar addiction. No support group you can go to, although there are increasing communities of support online. Because yes, it really is that difficult.

In addition to being processed differently by your body, fructose (the bit of sugar we're concerned with) plays games with your brain's ability to understand how much you've eaten and how hungry you are.

The general assumption goes like this. Years ago, when there were no man-made orchards or helpfully bagged-as-a-pack-of-six apples in easy reach, fruit was actually in pretty rare supply. And it's got a lot of good stuff in it that you'd want. It is also a great way of building up some extra fat to keep you going until you stumble across your next meal, or to get you through winter. It was never a huge part of the diet, so it wasn't something the body had to deal with in large quantities every day.

I could go deep into the biochemistry of leptin and grehlin and a whole load of other super-science words, but the bit you need to know for the purpose of your plan to become sugar-free is this:

- Fructose does not get 'seen' by your appetite regulation system as calories consumed
- Fructose helps stimulate more of the hormone that tells you that you're hungry

- Fructose also helps reduce the hormones that tell you that you're full and stop shoving that second cheeseburger in your mouth
- Fructose gives your brain a little 'high' and hardwires it to make you want more to get that high again

Those four key little facts about fructose are at the heart of why giving it up is so difficult and why we are consuming sugar and food in general in quantities greater than our bodies can cope with. Even when we know that it is in the food we are eating, the appetite control system that isn't part of our conscious brain isn't aware of it. That part of our body doesn't listen to the logical and knowing part of our mind. It simply doesn't register that you have consumed fructose and therefore it doesn't register the calories that are a part of it. The thing that it registers is a strange feeling that you want more. You're still feeling hungry in some curiously unsatisfied way, despite having consumed a large meal. Worse than unsatisfied, you find yourself actively craving more, despite being able to see that your stomach is bulging. The *feeling* is different to the reality.

Stack that all up and you can see why, despite

intellectually knowing all this, I've still fallen off the wagon so many times. Because, as with any kind of addiction, it takes a long time to unwire the brain. With sugar, there are dealers everywhere, on the supermarket shelves, in restaurants and certainly when you go to visit your friends and have to experience the additional social awkwardness of saying no and looking like a killjoy. Or smug and self-righteous, depending on how you play it. Neither is a good look regardless.

Understanding why your body is working against you, even in these hugely simplified ways is important, because the more you know, the more you'll understand what is happening when your body rebels. And it *will* rebel. Addiction is a horrible thing to go through. Ever tried quitting smoking? The dangers of smoking are hardly hidden. Cigarette packets these days practically reach out with their tiny arms to slap you in the face and yell *these are going to kill you!*, but it doesn't stop people lighting up.

So, from a realist's perspective, which is what this book promised to bring you, you are not going on a diet, you are breaking a significant addiction. This means a few things.

You *really* have to want to do it

Nobody ever half-heartedly breaks an addiction. I've yet to meet an alcoholic who sort of shrugged and said *it just happened* or *I didn't really think about it, just stopped fancying a drink.* I would even go out on a limb and say that if your goal is just to lose weight, then in the long term, that won't keep you sugar-free. Don't get me wrong, do it for a month, two months and you'll certainly lose weight. That much is pretty much guaranteed unless you deliberately sabotage yourself and continue eating even after you feel full. But keeping sugar-free in the face of daily temptation everywhere needs a stronger motivation than just losing ten pounds before you go to the beach for your summer holiday. My motivation? I want to be healthy, not just slim. I'm not going to lie and claim that size doesn't matter to me - I've grown up in the same world as everyone else with the same glossy magazine expectations - but skinny yet unhealthy isn't a place I want to be. I want to reduce the lifestyle damage I *can't* see. I want to be around for a long time, preferably living with my own internal organs, thank you very much.

There will be physical side effects

Sorry about that, but the whole point of this book is that I'm not going to lie to you, remember? I've read quite a few books about this and the majority of them tell you it will be hard for the first few days. They don't always explain what hard means. And the unspoken impression is that you just have to get through a few days and then *voila!* it will be easy from that point out.

Not so my friend.

In addition to the difficulty of having to use all your willpower not to reach for a chocolate bar, your body will experience withdrawal. Interestingly, and entirely anecdotally as far as I've been able to research - so I'm not even making any claims to basic science here - the length and impact of sugar-withdrawal seems to differ between men and women. Good news men! You seem to be able to give it up faster with weaker side effects. Ladies, your hormones seem to make it tougher. Like I said, entirely without any definitive research to back it up, as science doesn't care enough just yet. But any woman who would walk over hot coals and kick a puppy out of the way to get chocolate at a certain time of the month will know exactly what I mean.

Anyway, common side effects include:

- Headache
- Loss of concentration
- Flu-like symptoms
- Mood swings
- Exhaustion
- Trembling
- Anxiety and other mental health issues
- Insomnia

These are frequent side effects of any withdrawal process. Perhaps no one mentions them because that list is pretty off-putting. I'd rather you know in advance so you can be prepared. If you are already prone to any of those issues, then having a strategy in place to deal with them when they appear is much better than being taken by surprise when they suddenly get much worse for a day or three. For me, the headache and corresponding lack of concentration were the worst, which is probably why they appear at the top of my list.

For me, the first time I eliminated sugar went something a little like this...

Day 1 - Fuelled by determination and virtuousness about this whole sugar-free thing

Day 2 - Gratitude that I actually love salad anyway. This is going to be much easier. My willpower is STRONG

Day 3 - Why does my head hurt so much?

Day 4 - No, seriously, this is the worst headache I've ever had. Why hasn't it gone yet? Why am I peeing like a horse? I'm so sleepy. Please don't ask me to do anything that requires me to think

Day 5 - I TOLD YOU NOT TO ASK ME TO DO ANYTHING MY HEAD HURTS

Day 6 - Oooh, the pain is slightly less today. I just wish I didn't feel so tired, even if I did sleep properly last night for the first time in ages

Day 7 - I've made a week! Time to celebrate with some choco- Wait. No, can't do that. Hmmmm, this is really taking longer than I thought. When will I experience any joy in my life again? When?

Day 8 - Starting to feel a bit more human. Sudden realisation that this is just the beginning. I have to keep working harder for a while longer to maintain this...

That's just my recollection of events. I'm sure other people saw me as even more of a monster. It was tough. I did however monitor my daily calorie intake (in the name of pseudo-science) and it was roughly the same as it had been before I started the sugar-free approach. I did lose around 7lbs though, which at that point, was at least some incentive to keep going, even if it was probably just excess water.

You have been warned, so you can be prepared. Willpower alone is never enough...

You need a quitting plan in place

Everything I've written so far is not intended to demoralise you. I promise. It's to make you aware of all the little obstacles so you won't be surprised when they appear. Most of the success in embracing a sugar-free lifestyle comes not from the cooking itself, but from being prepared.

Decide when you're going to begin. Look at your calendar that week and make sure there are no high intensity activities you need to be present for - both physical *and* mental. Make sure there are no meals out with friends, kid's birthday parties or anything else where cake or a dessert menu will be practically obligatory. Be prepared to up your water intake. A lot. Bathrooms on hand are a must.

Approach it with grim determination. You are a warrior. You are about to do battle with your own body and your mind is likely to fail you midway through. Have a strategic plan in place and then follow it.

Another thing to consider is whether or not you've successfully quit anything addictive before. Or, on the opposite side of that coin, if you have successfully installed a new (hopefully good) habit, if quitting hasn't been your thing. Did you go cold turkey, or did you gently wean yourself away from/onto the habit? This could be useful in understanding which approach is most likely to result in success. I am one of those people who needs to go all out when doing anything. If I have the merest hint of the thing I am trying to avoid, then I relapse very quickly. Then I go the other way, into full on gluttonous excess for a few days. Other people have more success when slowly reducing things to limit the impact of any kind of addiction, which may be a better way forward for you. It is about *taking the time to think* about how you as an individual are most likely to succeed and then working with what you have. If you're not going to go cold turkey though, I will give you one word of warning. It is so easy to fool yourself that you are doing well because you gave up one thing. Sugar is so deeply immersed in our food world, giving up a single thing you perceive to be a naughty treat is not the same as making determined steps towards a sugar-free goal.

Final note on quitting: you *will* relapse

There will be times, no matter how good your intentions, no matter how much you understand the harm sugar does to your body, that you end up simply giving in and eating sugary processed food.

Sometimes, the decision will be all yours. It will be your birthday, or a holiday or you will simply have had a terrible day of work and the old habit of food reward will rear its head. Food is comforting. Especially the sweet stuff.

Other times, you may have no choice. Food preparation may be out of your control, such as when you go on holiday or if you're away at a conference and have to make the most of the hotel buffet three times a day.

So unless you're planning to live in a yurt, raise your

own livestock and grow your own crops, you're still going to have to live in this world. Chocolate is not suddenly going to disappear and neither is ketchup. Celebrations will still have food traditions attached. Food laced with sugar is going to cross your lips again at some point.

When this happens, be kind to yourself. Whether you relapse for one evening or if it's for a couple of weeks, that's not a reason to give up on being healthy for good. Surprisingly, you'll probably even find that once you've been off the sugar for a while, that after the initial high of going rogue, you'll feel pretty terrible. A week of normal, processed food and you'll feel bloated and sluggish. But the cravings will be back and you will have to learn to beat them again.

That's when you have to recommit, take a deep breath, focus, and climb back on the wagon. Believe that you can do it. By the end of this book, you'll know all the tips, tricks and tools to help you get back on your feet again.

CHAPTER THREE: SUGAR-FREE VS. OTHER DIETS

Why go sugar-free rather than one of the other diets?

Personally, as you've probably seen by now, I don't see going sugar-free as a 'diet'. That word alone comes with mental associations for most people. Negative associations, about feelings of lack, and hunger, and tasteless food and not enjoying yourself so you can be thin. When people say 'I'm going on a diet', those negatives are what the people they're telling think they mean and what, subconsciously, they often mean themselves.

It's a way of setting yourself up for failure. As humans, the majority of us don't tend towards masochism. We don't want to make ourselves suffer. So by embarking on anything that we believe is going to cause us pain or unhappiness on some level, we are going to be fighting against ourselves right from the start. We've already covered how your body is going to rebel against you anyway, so take that 'diet' barrier out of your head. Consider it, instead, as a lifestyle change. A new habit to build a stronger, healthier you.

The beauty of going sugar-free is that once you've removed it from your system, it no longer messes with those 'I'm hungry/I'm full' hormones. So as long as you're not eating sugar, you never have to think about calories again.

Imagine that: *never worrying about calories again.*

Quite simply, when your body has consumed the food it needs, it tells you. I've eaten a giant steak with loads of vegetables for dinner and not found myself hungry again until after lunchtime the following day. I didn't have breakfast because I wasn't hungry. It's a brave new world, but it's actually easier than trying to gauge the size of your potato to work out how many calories it contains.

Sugar-free vs. Calorie Controlled/Points systems

There are other very well known approaches to building a newer, healthier you that are built around essentially controlling your calories. Corporate global diet schemes where you weigh in once a week and buy a lot of branded products. To me, those aren't even comparable to this. Often you have to maintain a set number of calories or points a day, or have days when you have to think about restricting your food to a very narrow group that may still contain multiple artificial products. People *do* lose weight on these diets. A calorie deficit will indeed lead to weight loss. However, a strict calorie restriction often leads to a plateau that many find disheartening. Again, this is simple evolution: your metabolic system slows down because you've entered the metaphorical dessert. Your body does its best to become even more efficient, holding onto and storing every unit of energy it can to allow you to survive until you've made it through the wilderness.

From a health perspective, we've already established that skinny doesn't equal healthy anyway. Often those branded products contain all kinds of chemical nasties, not just excessive amounts of sugar. The goal in this instance is actually only about convincing weight loss, not long-term health benefits. Being sugar-free means that real, sustainable weight loss happens naturally, without any of the constant monitoring and without long-term feelings of hunger. Most importantly, it happens without putting damaging products into your system for the primary purpose of staying within your points/calories for the day.

Sugar-free vs. Carb-free

Going ultra low carb means by default you'll be going sugar-free. So if you prefer this option, then good for you. If you go low carb, you'll definitely seem more of an impact on your weight. This is why the low carb diet has long been the choice of the ultra-healthy and those into serious fitness. It is very effective. The downside? It is much harder to maintain and unless you *really* understand what is going on underneath, you can get massively demoralised if you have a 'bad' day.

Your whole body works differently when you're on ultra low carb. It is a state you need to maintain a lot more, because your body will then instantly cling to any carbs you eat on your bad day. Unfortunately, in order to cling to that energy source and top up your fully depleted glycogen stores as a result, it needs to bind itself to a lot of water. A lot of heavy, heavy water. So a single bad day can cost you an instant 5lb gain on the scales. If you understand how that works and it is part of your plan, then you'll know that as you get back to normal, that energy will get used and the excess water thrown away again very quickly. If you *don't* understand how it works, and you are doing it to 'diet' then you'll quickly find yourself demoralised and lose the mental game. It is very easy to then get into the mindset of 'whenever I eat anything nice I put a load of weight straight on' and that very quickly spirals to 'what's the point'. That's a hop, skip and jump to giving up and sitting in front of the TV with a tub of ice cream.

So if you are just looking to get your body to a sensible weight and maintain it, the sugar-free option is more feasible as an approach. It's nice to think that the diet of ultra-athletes is the one for us, but unless you really have that dedication and focus, going carb-free becomes very difficult to sustain. The beauty of sugar-free instead is that it will automatically lower your carb intake to a sensible (but not near zero) level, so you get a lot of the same health benefits. Without sugar messing with your brain, your body will see those carbs and let you know when you've had enough of them, so you can stop eating to excess more effectively than before.

If you've tried low carb before and ended up craving bread so much that you quit, then sugar-free is more likely to work for you. Carbs are allowed and as long as you know what to look for (see the shopping section later), you don't even need to go to the hassle of baking your own. There are also some studies indicating that ketosis (the name for the state your body goes into when completely deprived of carbohydrates) is not great for long-term health either.

Sugar-free vs. Paleo

There are several versions of the 'Paleolithic Diet' around, geared towards different levels of dedication and intensity. But the basic principles of *could I have eaten this in my cave 50,000 years ago?* apply. By this definition it automatically excludes processed foods, so there is definitely some overlap between the two approaches. There is a similar heavy emphasis on meat, vegetables, fruits and nuts, so again, by doing the Paleo diet (unless you over-emphasise fruit) you will also by default become largely sugar-free.

As with low carb, there is an element of dedication required that makes Paleo difficult to sustain over the long term for many people. As well as cutting out processed foods, there are several other assumptions around what edible products were available to us when we didn't have to wash and the only thing on our to do list was to kill a buffalo, then find a wall so we could paint a picture about it. We didn't yet do anything with the buffalo, such as milk it, before we killed it to eat, so dairy is off the list. So are grains, widely introduced into some diets when farming began at around 15,000BC, but not before. Legumes (known as things like peas, beans, lentils to you and me) are out as well. The list is getting narrower. No salt for flavour and no alcohol to take away the misery of what you're doing.

Plus the final straw that stopped me from ever, *ever* considering this diet: no coffee.

By all accounts (again, there isn't masses of research yet to back this up), people with certain food intolerances can really benefit from going Paleo. If that's you and the health benefits outweigh eating or drinking those restricted foods, then by all means, head down the Paleo route. If you don't have those intolerances, or they're so mild they don't really factor into your daily life, then it comes down to sustainability. Like the ultra-low carb approach, there is an element of dedication required to stay on this diet that makes avoiding sugar - which as we've discovered is no small feat in itself - look significantly easier in comparison.

Seriously, no coffee? How do people on Paleo even get up in the morning?

Anyway, that is how sugar-free stacks up with some

of the other well known, similar approaches. It has several advantages, but for me, long-term sustainability once you get past your addiction is the key. Still on board with this whole lifestyle change? Then it's probably time to begin.

CHAPTER FOUR: HABIT TRACKING

This might seem like an odd place to start. Most 'diet' books start with food. They follow with exercise, if you really want to make the most of the benefits and *get that bikini body fast!*

I'll keep hammering this point home: this little book is meant to be realistic and help you go sugar-free over the long term. To do that, we have to go deeper and look at the foundations of what makes it possible to achieve this: habits.

As I pointed out with the alternative diets, sustainability when living in a highly constricted way is always very difficult. You need to have a particular level of focus and dedication. Those who succeed at maintaining this level of self control usually have two things going for them: a purpose (athletic body, avoiding food intolerances etc) and discipline. I can't tell you what your purpose is, but I can tell you what underpins discipline, and that is habit.

Chances are that you will have some existing bad habits with food. We all do. Mine, for example, come in the form of Friday night treats to celebrate the start of the weekend and Sunday night commiseration food when I realise it's over. Holidays are another time when I relax and stop thinking about everything in any way that could be even remotely considered as disciplined. Swapping to sugar-free, especially when you add in the addiction to the white stuff itself, is going to require you to break those habits. Or, as a better way of doing it, replace them with new ones.

The problem with habits is that they are unconscious. It doesn't matter whether it is a good behaviour or a bad behaviour, once it becomes a habit we do it on autopilot and our brain ceases to question whether it is the *right* thing to do in that moment. So tackling this problem needs conscious thought to get the old habits out and the new habits in. The good news? Conscious thought and effort in advance is much more likely to work and, in many ways is easier, than simply willpowering your way through the entire process. So, the first step in becoming sugar-free is to life hack your day.

Define your habits

Along with everything else in this book, honest and realistic are the watch words. If you are interested in going sugar-free enough to have read this far, then you owe it to yourself to set yourself up for success, no matter how uncomfortable that may be in the short term.

There is a good chance that consuming sugar and the feel good high you get immediately after are tied to a set of habits that occur. One thing to remember is that the vast majority of alcoholic drinks contain significant amounts of sugar. So if you're one of those people who have a certain tipple at a certain time, you need to include that too. I am not going to touch on alcoholism in this book (as it is a topic far bigger than I have either the space or capacity to cover), but if you find yourself feeling an uncomfortable pull when faced with the prospect of giving up your daily drink habit, then you may want to seek advice for that elsewhere too.

Another critical success factor here is to write each habit down as you go along. On paper, they will feel much more real. Work your way through each of the days of the week and their corresponding times of the day (just morning, afternoon and evening will do unless you really want to get into the detail, in which case, knock yourself out, the more the better). You'll probably find at least two or three key times of the week when a food 'treat' is a given. I'm going to go out on a limb and say that the food treat you choose turns out to be a salad approximately zero per cent of the time. Whether you are a sweet or a savoury person by nature will affect what you think of as a treat, but remember that a pizza and a beer could contain as much sugar as a latte and a slice of cake.

Now expand your thinking beyond that. Are there key events that are likely to be sugar heavy? The obvious ones are holidays or birthdays if you celebrate them. There are many religious events, regardless of which particular belief system you follow, which celebrate with a feast. What began as a symbol of gratitude and thanks for abundance provided has become an excuse to gorge ourselves on all the food we can fit in until we feel uncomfortable enough to undo a few buttons. These events are not going to go away just because you've decided to eliminate sugar from your life. You can't just ignore them, so be *aware* of them. That way you can plan to minimise the damage without alienating all of your family and friends. Unless you've been looking for an excuse for years to avoid those occasions, in which case this might be it. You're welcome!

The good news is that the longer you spend on the sugar-free lifestyle and the more other people become aware of it, the less they buy you chocolate. Someone still will though, because the 'celebration and food' approach is a habit for them too. Either that or they're too lazy to come up with something else. You can be as generous as you like in your opinion as to which is the case in your own family.

Knowledge is power

Once you have defined your bad habits and the times/days they are likely to occur, you have two ways to fight – and beat - them. The first is that you can prepare for them and the second is that you can replace them with something else.

Preparation is good when food challenges are tied into an unmovable event, like a holiday or celebration. Instead of stumbling thoughtlessly into the room and having to watch other people eat while your stomach growls and protests, you can find an alternative approach. Let's face it, if you turn up hungry to something where there are no sugar-free choices, your willpower is unlikely to be sufficient when the cake is placed in front of you. Willpower is massively overrated and useless for most of us when faced with something like this. You cannot make the event bend to your will, so either eat beforehand or cheerfully bring an alternative that works for you (if that is possible and won't offend your host).

If you're going to a restaurant, most of them have a menu online these days. Check it out beforehand and find the sugar-free options. Chances are, you'll be limited to very few choices and might even have to just go for the best option available and take the hit. But make a decision *there and then,* in the comfort of your home when the appearance of food isn't actually imminent. Then when you get there, don't look at the menu again. Seriously. Looking again will no doubt undo all your good intentions. If your friends are like mine, they'll probably read aloud most of the tasty-but-terrible-for-you sounding options, turning it into some kind of casual torture session. Do not engage. Do not look down to see what they are talking about so that it becomes a temptation. Humans are terrible with temptation and you are no exception. Make a decision beforehand, close your ears and stick to your order when the waiter or waitress comes round.

It may be hard to believe now, but when the dessert menu comes round, the longer you've been sugar-free, the easier it is to say no. This is not because you become some kind of Jedi master of willpower, although you can feel better about yourself by believing that if you wish. It's because your body resets, like we talked about earlier, letting you know when you really have consumed enough by making you feel properly full. Even sugar-free meals in restaurants and pubs tend to be on the large side of portion control, so you will actually start to feel pleasantly stuffed and unable to fit in dessert after your main meal. You can always order a coffee instead if other people are eating, and I've yet to find myself in a situation where someone else won't take the biscotti or mint on the side if it comes with one.

For slightly more everyday events, then preparation isn't your only option, but it is certainly valid. If you absolutely can't break your Friday night takeaway habit, then do your research beforehand and switch to something that is sugar-free or really low sugar. There are little tricks you can do, like adding extra fibre to the meal to slow the absorption of any extra sugar into your system, giving your liver a better chance and reducing the impact of the blood sugar spike. As with restaurant meals, the principles remain the same: do the decision-making beforehand, when you've got a clear and logical head. When faced with making a decision in the moment, you'll more than likely make the wrong one. When shopping (more on that later), buy things such as popcorn (not sweet, obviously) that *feel* like a treat, without actually breaking the rules. Then if you find yourself unconsciously walking to the kitchen cupboards (this is a habit remember, so chances are you won't even realise you're doing it until the door is open and you're buried halfway inside rummaging around on the shelves for a snack), all the options you pull out won't be too damaging.

Where possible, the best solution is not to just break the habit, but to replace it with another. See this as a golden opportunity to do something you always wanted to do. This doesn't have to be big. I'm not saying you need to take up Tango dancing or triathlons. You don't have to go out and invest in an easel and paints because you want to stop eating a Mars bar. It can be as simple as taking the time to start reading more rather than watching TV (a prime time for bad habit snacking) or making a list of the small odd jobs around the house you've been putting off for the last decade and then ticking off one each week. If you replace the bad eating habit time with something that gives you a little positive boost of either enjoyment or achievement, you're much more likely to get the momentum to keep going. That will become your new habit and pretty soon, you'll stop having to think about it and just do it, like you did with food and drink before.

Finally, track your good days and get a sense of reward. There are many ways of doing this, depending on your personal preference. I use a habit tracking app on my phone, but a lot of people use pen and paper. The key is to *give yourself a visual representation* of how many days you've been sugar-free. See how long you can go without breaking the chain. Once you get to a certain point, filling your tick box in every day, your naturally competitive and reward-driven brain will kick in. You'll find yourself thinking about the number of days in a row you've done already and if you do have that slice of pizza or cake you'll be forced back to zero. It has an amazing power. The only caveat is this: if you do break the streak, it is not an excuse to just stop and give up. One slip up, or one event that you simply can't get out of and had no choice but to consume food that is not on your plan, does not mean that the next day you do the same again. Acknowledge it, be kind to yourself and then go into the following day determined to get that first checkbox completed again.

As I mentioned earlier, you will slip up. There may be whole days which don't go your way, or even longer than that. Having a slice of cake does not mean you've failed. Get that defeatist mindset out of your head right now. Failure is giving up and allowing bad health to ultimately limit something you want from your life. Instead, change your habits, change your future.

At the end of this book, you'll find space to write down your habits before you begin, as well as example habit trackers to use during the first month.

CHAPTER FIVE: HOW TO GO SHOPPING

So far, like an annoying parent or troublesome teacher, I've spent most of this telling you all the things you can't do. We're one step away from me sending you to your room and grounding you for the weekend.

Now we can get onto the one thing you probably thought you were going to be reading about right from the start. It is time to talk about the food you *can* have.

Sugar is used as a preservative and flavour enhancer in just about everything. The nutrition labels on food globally are improving all the time and at least you can see these things now. Many countries still use carbohydrates as a single value, without breaking it down into sugars. This can be unhelpful as we're not trying to avoid all carbs on this diet.

The alternative way is to look at the list of ingredients and see if sugar is on there. If it is, scrap it from the list. Also, consider yourself lucky to have found it; something with a clearly worded *sugar* is a quick victory against the food industry.

I've created a fake nutrition label below for a tasty Asian sauce. By fake, I mean 'hopefully won't get me sued by a big food conglomerate' rather than 'inaccurate'. I've highlighted the key features in **bold**.

NUTRITION FACTS	
INGREDIENTS	
Water, **Sugar**, **Glucose-Fructose Syrup**, Soy Sauce [Water, Salt, **Sugar**, Barley Malt Extract, Defatted Soya Bean Flakes, Colour (Plain Caramel), Yeast Extract, Spirit Vinegar, Wheat], Modified Maize Starch, Onion Purée, Ginger Purée, Spring Onion, Garlic Purée, Garlic Powder, Red Chilli Peppers, Salt, Acetic Acid, Sesame Oil, Yeast Extract Paste, Acidity Regulator (Citric Acid)	
Typical Values	Typical Values per 100 g
Energy	436 kJ / 103 kcal
Fat	0.9 g
of which saturates	0.1 g
Carbohydrate	24 g
of which sugars	**16 g**
Protein	0.8 g
Salt	1.6 g

Sugar and a syrup are in the top three ingredients,

and sugar is also a component of the soy sauce. So it is easy to see how the 'of which sugars' part of the carbohydrates are well above the 5g per 100g (5%) that serves as a good cut off figure.

I recently looked at the ingredients of a low fat, 'light' cereal bar, designed to be ideal for snacking mid morning. It had less than 70 calories, which put it firmly in the 'good' camp when looking at things the traditional way you've probably been used to. Also less than a gram of fat, which is the other thing we've always been taught to look out for. Fabulous. Throw that in the basket if you want to lose weight, right?

Wrong.

It might not have any fat, but it had nearly 5 grams of sugar. We've been aiming at sugar-free (max 10g/day) so far, but for women, current guidelines indicate that you should consume no more than 25g of sugar per day (35g for men). Given this number is now under scrutiny and may itself be too high, acting simply as a guideline deemed to be achievable - rather than actually healthy - for most people, there is a chance it could get lowered. Let us pretend for now though it is acceptable. In that case ladies, the cereal bar which tasted like pleasantly sweet air and left you feeling quite empty an hour later, was a 20% hit into your daily allowance. That's a significant percentage for something so tiny. How can this be?

This is where looking at the label comes back in. To understand anything of what you are consuming these days, you need to become a master of the ingredients labelling.

I never said being healthy was going to be glamorous. That's what those other books are for, remember?

In the low fat cereal bar example above, in order to produce something that was low in calories, low in fat but didn't taste like it was sweepings from a factory floor, something needed to be added. A lot of somethings in fact.

To make that bar of delicious nothingness, it took thirty-three ingredients. Many of which would give you fantastic word scores in scrabble because they use all kinds of letters that don't get seen together outside of chemistry. The words most people *would* understand seem healthy enough, things like 'apple' and 'cranberry'. Sadly, those fruits are mentioned in the context of fruit concentrate, which is just a way to get the sugar out of them and very little else of nutritional benefit. Thirteen of the thirty three ingredients were sugar additions and whether it originated from a fruit once (probably a very long time ago in the factory process) or is a complete chemical composition, your body doesn't care. A simple check is does the word end in *-ose?* Fructose, dextrose, oligofructose (a personal favourite), all of these are ways of adding in sweetness. Our bodies like sweet and food manufacturers know it.

It is not until you start looking for sugar and its sweet chemical companions that you begin to realise just how many strange ingredients there are in our food. Children's foods that are promoted as healthy are just as bad. If you notice the way food is marketed, it only ever promotes what it *doesn't* contain. It tricks the average shopper, usually with not a lot of time to browse, into picking it up and throwing it in the basket because it doesn't contain a specific item they've previously been warned about. *Less than 1% fat!* is a much more grabbing headline than *so many preservatives this bar will survive nuclear fallout!* Unless a Cold Winter is somewhere in your future or you're actively planning for a zombie apocalypse, then you don't need that at your desk when you're surfing emails at 11am.

Given that single small example, it is impossible for

the average person to look at every single item of food they would normally buy as part of their weekly shopping trip and work out what is in it. It would be utterly demoralising, plus you'd be that person who moves through the aisles so slowly they block the whole thing up and everyone hates them (you know who I'm talking about). It's much better to start out with some rules that allow you to move quickly through the shopping experience and out the other side with your sanity still intact.

As sugar is added to most processed foods, the logical place to start is with unprocessed foods. Genius, right? Yet it isn't until you actively *start* doing it that you realise how little of those you were putting in before.

Assuming you're not vegetarian, meat is your first obvious choice. Sugar-free by nature, it's completely allowed. If you can go organic, even better, but for a lot of people, the cost is off-putting and I understand that. There have been several health warnings about 'processed' meats, such as bacon, or red meats such as beef, hitting the headlines in recent years. If you only care about being sugar-free, then a good quality bacon is on the list. If you want to be more health conscious in general, then you can consider swapping to a white meat and fish. Your personal preferences on meat are not going to be dictated by me.

Assuming you are allowing all meats in, then don't fall into the trap of buying pre-packaged cooked meats. A significant number of these either come with delicious flavourings (sugar) or have been packaged for a longer shelf life (sugar). This can be hard to navigate, as many of these meats have been carved from the deli counter do not come in packaging with labels, leaving you almost entirely in the dark about added ingredients. If you're not sure, then do not put it into the basket.

Fruit and vegetables come next and again, this is fair game across the board. A lot of people get confused about fruit when deciding to become sugar-free. After all, we are trying to avoid fructose and it got its name from its naturally occurring nature in fruit. One piece per day is absolutely fine, as long as you eat the actual whole fruit. Not fruit as a juice, not fruit preserved in concentrate, not fruit in a smoothie (although many of these are significantly better than a juice). If the fruit still looks exactly the same as when it was growing, then you're fine.

However, fruit juices and smoothies are promoted to us as healthy. In a world where it is hard to get our five a day, it is a quick fix. Who doesn't love a palatable shortcut? Sadly, this is in many ways just another clever marketing attempt. Fruit, whilst naturally containing fructose, also contains a lot of natural fibre. Fibre has the impact of slowing down how your body processes sugar and makes it much kinder to your liver. It also fills you up, to prevent you from gorging on the fruit. If you want to avoid sweet fruit altogether, that is fine, as long as you're eating plenty of vegetables instead. But do not make the mistake of drinking juices that have had the fibre removed and the sugar increased. A glass of orange juice has only one to two grams of sugar less than a glass of cola and your body needs to process it in exactly the same way. You might as well take a vitamin tablet with a can of soda. A single large glass could blow your recommended sugar intake for the entire day and you'd probably drink it in only a couple of minutes. That is a lot for your liver to have to deal with and it's just going to pump out those fatty acids we're trying to avoid. Smoothies, whilst having the benefit of some fibre remaining, can contain even more sugar than juices. If it doesn't look like it did when it was on the tree, then tread with caution. This goes for dried fruit too. Deliciously sweet and compact so you can eat even more, they are little pellets of sugar in convenient packaging. Those handy child friendly boxes contain around 70% sugar, coming in at a whopping 25g.

Vegetables, fresh or frozen, are allowed. Simple as that. Canned may come with preservatives and other nasties, so they should be avoided if possible. Plus, one less aisle to have to walk down.

Now, I'm not foolish enough to believe that you'll be eating nothing but chicken and vegetables whilst living in your commune and drinking pure mountain spring water. So what about other food? When it comes to shopping, here's a quick and by no means comprehensive guide, but it will give you a good enough place to start.

Dairy

Again, I'm writing this from the assumption that you're not vegan or intolerant to dairy products. If you are, then I have very little experience of non-dairy alternatives other than to note that many 'dairy style' options have added sugar to make them more palatable. Always double check the label. If you're going to exclude dairy altogether, then you should consult a doctor or nutritionist to ensure you still get the positive nutritional benefits they usually provide.

So, dairy products in their pure form are your friend on the sugar-free diet. Ignoring anything fancy, like the recent penchant for adding fruit and odd flavourings, cheese is a good option. When I was starting sugar-free, someone recommended that when I got the sweet cravings in the evening, I should just eat a cube of cheese. No crackers, just the cheese. I have no idea why it works, but it does. This is particularly useful when starting out and the sweet cravings come frequently.

However - no processed cheeses! If the look and feel of the end product is closer to something you would find in a plastics factory than the milk it came from, then that's generally a good sign something has been done to it that you don't want anywhere near your body. Many UK/USA processed cheeses contain stabilisers and preservatives that are banned in other parts of the world, such as Australia and New Zealand. Cheese slices and triangles are the obvious culprits, although it should be noted that the actual cheese/preservative content varies by brand. Check the label: if there are more than three ingredients, then avoid it if you can.

Speaking of milk, it is the most obvious dairy product and probably should have come first on this list, but I'm a cheesaholic so it didn't occur to me to make it a top priority. For the rest of you relatively normal people, milk is probably more of interest in your daily lives. Again, this is one of those strange areas where in many countries, skimmed or fat-free milk has been pushed on us for decades as the sensible choice to make. The last time I regularly had full fat milk was as a child, when a man on a milk float was still delivering it in fat little bottles with silver foil lids. Yet whole milk is only 3-4% fat. Of all the products that pushed so hard to be low fat for very little gain, this has to be the winner. Low fat milk contains more sugar, although much of this will be the milk sugars (lactose) that some people are intolerant to. Lactose, if you remember from our whirlwind tour of sugar types earlier, is not the problem here. Our bodies are very much aware of lactose and handle it in a different way to the sugar (fructose) we are trying to avoid here. If you *are* intolerant, you'll know just how differently...

Ahem. Moving on.

It goes without saying; flavoured milk is not an option. A strange health gamble designed to appeal to kids and adults alike, flavoured milk often has copious amounts of added sugar to make it taste deliciously fruity or chocolatey. Once you've been sugar-free for a while, you'll notice that milk has a slight, naturally sweet taste anyway. It's just masked under our current expectations of how sweet our addicted bodies like things to be.

The other obvious dairy product for the dieter has always been yoghurt. Sadly, for most normal people, yoghurt tastes absolutely disgusting. It's sour and tangy and feels very unpleasant in your mouth. Greek yoghurt is the taste of yoghurt and most of the time people who eat that add either fruit or honey to stop their eyes from watering. However, you can strip out the fat and replace it with sugar to make a highly marketable diet product that is low fat and actually tastes quite nice.

As you've probably worked out by now, if something is labelled either healthy or low fat, it's probably the very worst thing you can have. I'll give props to chocolate; at least it doesn't lie about what it is. Yoghurt, on the other hand, is one of the biggest health slight-of-hand tricks that has ever been pulled. A low fat yoghurt can have up to 18g of sugar per serving (that's the highest I've found in my very unscientific mooch around the shelves before I got bored and depressed). That's the same as in, wait for it, 6 digestive biscuits (or 4 and a bit regular

Oreos, for my American readers).

If you're going to have yoghurt, have full fat, natural, unsweetened, unflavoured yoghurt. Sweeten it with fruit (whole) if you like, but not honey. It might be one of nature's sweeteners, but it's still sugar and having it will just make it harder to quit and easier to begin that backwards slide.

Finally, use butter. We don't care about fat on this diet, because our bodies learn how to recognise it again. But more importantly, low fat spreads and margarines can contain anything. For years, trans fats and other nasties were added to our foods without understanding the consequences. At least if you only use butter, you know that the next chemically created fat substitute they suddenly admit to being damaging to human health won't be an issue for you. There are other fat alternatives, such as coconut oil of course, but you won't find them in the dairy section, which is why I'll specifically refer to butter in this instance.

Bread

Many people believe if you're going to go sugar-free, then you need to stop eating bread. Not so! I'm not going to be that cruel to you.

Many people seem to struggle on the ultra-low carb diet with the horrible reality of not being able to eat bread specifically. After all, what is the point of being allowed unlimited bacon if you can't wedge it between two slices? Sugar-free allows you to have some bread and this is one of the things that makes the diet manageable long term for me.

When looking for bread on the supermarket shelves, skip straight past the processed white stuff. Almost every diet tells you not to have that. However, once you get to the less fun bread, you still need to tread with caution. Why? For the simple reason that bread manufacturers are just as clever as every other type of food marketer.

Brown, wholemeal, whole-wheat, any other healthy sounding named bread actually doesn't taste that great, especially when you're switching from white. Depending on the base recipe, manufacturers know this and just like the 'low fat' branding, will only tell you the parts that are marketable. So 'high in fibre' 'made from whole wheat' is what they'll splash across the front, not *tastes pretty rough, so we added some sugar so you can actually swallow it.*

Yes, they add sugar into brown bread, often in

greater quantities than white bread. I did warn you right at the start that sugar was sneaky and could get in just about anywhere.

So, when looking for a loaf of bread, make sure the sugars are still very low, preferably 1g or less per slice. Most importantly, as a counter balance, make sure *that the fibre is really high*. Fibre is nature's counterbalance remember, that slows down how quickly our body gets its sugar hit when we eat, so aim for 2.5g or more per slice. Low sugar, high fibre bread exists and you can have a couple of slices a day without breaking the sustainable 'sugar-free' lifestyle we're trying to achieve here.

In a similar vein, not all carbohydrates are off limits. Wholewheat pasta, couscous and wholewheat noodles can all be found in relatively low sugar (less than 3%) varieties. Just don't buy any pre-flavoured ones, as these can add several grams of sugar per serving.

Seasonings

Of course, with all of this 'straight from the field' food, you're going to want to make it actually taste good. After years of having flavour overload, to go completely without would be a huge shock to the system. The good news is that herbs, spices, salt and pepper are all excellent. Throw in as much as you want (with the exception of salt, which I'll talk about more at the end of this chapter). Be creative.

What you don't want to use are pre-packaged seasoning mixes. They are convenient, yes, I won't deny that. In the modern world, we have reached a point where having to add spices from four different jars seems akin to a level of culinary complexity that only top chefs can achieve. Not to mention time consuming. However, that convenience is paid for in the added sugar. A single quick example that hammers the point home: a delicious and well known fajita seasoning mix contains, wait for it, *50% sugar*. That is not a typo. It is literally half a packet of sugar you are adding to your strips of chicken and beef to get that spicy BBQ flavour. Don't do it.

Commercial mayonnaise has sugar added to it (of course) and ketchup of all kinds becomes taboo. Despite assuming before I started this I had a relatively healthy diet, I was probably feeding my sugar addiction with ketchup alone. My regular brand was 28% sugar and I'm fairly certain that what I squeezed onto my plate wasn't what they classed as a single serving. Add that to the delicious low fat cereal bar I'd had mid afternoon and the low fat yoghurt I'd had for lunch and my blood was swimming in sugar-induced fatty acids without even trying.

Many herbs and spices have been traditionally used because of the health benefits they provide. Science is now backing up many old wives' tales on this and therefore you have nothing to lose by using them. It's not actually as hard as it looks and once you find something you like, it becomes really easy to use every day.

Seeds and nuts

Once we get into the realms of seeds and nuts it all starts to sound a bit more like a traditional fanatical health kick. Knowing the latest unpronounceable grain from some far-off region that has miracle health properties is a level I'm not willing to go to. But seeds and nuts do have their uses and have been long neglected in modern cooking.

If you have a nut allergy, then please do not follow this advice. If you don't, then buy mixed packs to snack on. Go for as wide a variety as you can, because different nuts bring all kinds of things to the table. Once you're sugar-free, a handful of nuts actually does become enough, which is something I never thought would be the case back when I could shovel dry roasted peanuts down my throat by the actual handful (yes, I know a peanut isn't actually a nut, but clearly that's not the point I'm trying to make here). As always, whole nuts, unflavoured are the way to go. They're pretty easy to transport around for snack purposes too, which adds a convenience factor worth mentioning.

Did you say seeds? Like, the stuff birds eat?

Before I started my quest to be sugar-free, my natural response to the suggestion of seeds would indeed have been 'seeds are for birds'. To be honest, that's still my primary response, but you can't expect me to change overnight. Seeds have a huge part to play in living a healthy lifestyle and because they don't have any of the glamorous marketing element or super convenience factor, they've dropped further down the list of things that humans eat. However, this book is a start up guide, not really for those who are already health nuts (every pun intended). If you are already incorporating seeds into your diet then good for you. You're doing it right and keep going. For everyone else, my one tip would be to buy a bag of linseed (or flaxseed as it is sometimes labelled) and start there. Why? Because it doesn't taste of anything in particular so you won't find your taste buds offended first thing in the morning and because it contains nearly 30% fibre. That means not only will it help slow down its own (very small) sugar content, it will slow down that of everything else as well. Besides which, everyone knows they're not getting enough fibre in their diets these days, contributing to all kinds of long term health issues, but it's always really hard to find it in packaged products so we constantly struggle to get any better at consuming it. A couple of spoons of linseed on your breakfast cereal in the morning is barely noticeable and will set your body up right for the day. Speaking of breakfast cereal...

Breakfast Cereal

Why does breakfast cereal get a whole section of its own when it's not exactly a food group? Quite simply, it is one of the most dangerous areas for those beginning sugar-free. It deserves a special warning all of its own.

For years, breakfast has been pushed as the most important meal of the day. There have been numerous claims that those who lose the most weight on a diet, or those who are thinnest to begin with, eat breakfast. I'm not going to dispute that. I am merely going to point out that breakfast cereals clearly do not fall into the type of food that our ancestors picked up as they were crossing the plains looking for their next meal and evolving our biology into the efficient food consuming machine it is today. We are not the pinnacle of evolution (or god's highest creation, if you choose to see if that way) because our purpose in life was to be able to consume flakes with extra frosting from a box with a cartoon on it.

Again, this is one of the areas I am most passionate about because so much of it is aimed towards children. Getting children to eat breakfast has been a marketing success story. Yet it is often starting them off with a significant amount of sugar whilst claiming it to be healthy, just because it has been fortified with a few minerals and some iron. As you pull that box out of the cupboard with the smiling cartoon character of your choice, know that what makes breakfast so appealing to you and your kids is up to 40% sugar. Not actually a great way to start your day, no matter how palatable. Also explains why you're hungry again by 10:30 for that matter, doesn't it?

I'm sure there are people reading this who feel a tad virtuous on the matter of breakfast, as they eat 'healthy' cereals only. The ones aimed at those who believe they are sophisticated adults rather than overworked mums just desperately trying to get their kids to eat something so they won't be late for school. Again. People for whom breakfast is muesli or granola because it sounds like a mature and healthy start to the day. Generally, the adverts for this have a woman wearing sportswear all fired up for a great day ahead, or perhaps a natural country feel to make you believe this is how breakfast used to be in the good old days, depending on which brand you choose.

What have we learned about things marketed as healthy by now folks? Guess what? These are actually some of the absolute worst when it comes to sugar content. Often they only add natural sugars (marketing alert!), but of course, these all come from concentrated fruit. Most of them contain fruit, because, honestly, why else would you eat those floor sweepings in the first place, right? I've found some around the 40% sugar mark, which is an impressive hit to start your day with, especially when you consider that, by density, you'll probably consume a greater weight of product than those fluffy children's cereals. As I write this, I have noticed that many of them seem to be slowly reducing their sugar content or introducing lower sugar versions of their original products, so there is some hope for the future. But for sugar-free, stick to a good wholemeal toast – no jam, obviously - or, if at all possible, bacon/steak/ham and eggs. A full protein approach will keep you fuller for longer and won't start your day off with a massive sugar spike that you then spend all day combating the effects of. Shredded Wheat is about the only cereal I've found that contains no added sugar, so that gets the thumbs up from me if you really must have pre-packaged cereals. Throw some seeds and blueberries on there and you can feel genuinely smug and virtuous.

What about artificial sweeteners?

For many people, this is the truly grey area when embarking on the sugar-free lifestyle. After so many years of consuming sugar and developing the taste for it, how can we make things taste palatable enough to stay away for long enough that we actually break the addiction?

Again, it comes down to your habits and how you like to do things. The long term benefits and risks of chemical sugar alternatives aren't really known and some of the compounds seem to be a little bit dubious. However, in the short term, they might be what you need to get that little bit of sweet flavour to not fall straight back off the wagon.

When I started out my own journey into sugar-free, I attempted using some of these artificial sweeteners so I could bake without everything tasting utterly, utterly wrong. It didn't exactly make my muffins culinary delights to be proud of, but most of them were at least edible. After about a month of being sugar-free, all I could taste was a slightly chemical effect once I'd eaten them. By then, I was losing the taste for sweetness anyway, so giving up sweet treats - however flavoured - was becoming a bit easier. So whilst I don't like the thought of using artificial sweeteners long term in my own diet, I can certain see the benefits of using them as a gentle stepping stone towards losing that craving and taste for sugar in the short term. Anything to make the process that little bit easier is worth considering.

A word on salt

Given that this approach to nutrition is to avoid fructose, it stands to reason that you'll replace sweet items with more savoury ones. From my own experience, it became very easy to increase my salt intake as a result. You can find a significant number of crisps (chips for my American readers), pretzel pieces and meat-based snacks that contain significantly high levels of salt. The impact of salt on high blood pressure, amongst other things has been well documented over the years. Many successful campaigns have been led to get people to reduce their salt intake and low salt versions of food have been around long before their low sugar counterparts were even considered. So do not replace one unhealthy additive with another. Enjoy savoury snacks, but don't live on them. As with anything in life, you can cheat the system, but in the long run, you're only cheating yourself.

So now you have a shopping basket filled with fresh vegetables, fruits and meat, some herbs and spices and maybe some cheese and eggs. Nothing processed and brightly marketed as a health food, messing with your mind (as well as your body) as you go. What next? Well, next is the hard part for a lot of people.

You have to learn to cook, and preferably enjoy doing so...

CHAPTER SIX: LEARN TO LOVE COOKING

If you actually enjoy cooking and have ample time to do it, then congratulations, you have a head start. I strongly suspect most people reading this won't fall into that category.

Cooking has become something of luxury in modern society. In some western countries, there is the simple fact you can go out for noodles or pizza at the same cost as buying the ingredients for a meal, without losing the time to prepare it yourself. Eating is also sociable; you can join your friends and get two things done at once. I understand that. I am not going to be able to make those decisions for you about whether the cost saving in time is worth the detriment to your health. We see the effects of that calculation and trade off in rising obesity rates everywhere. Children are increasingly having their own spending power and are buying into tasty convenience as well. The problem isn't going to go away unless we do something about it.

The good news is that cooking can be a social activity too. If that is your excuse for going out to eat, then inviting your friends over for dinner has two benefits; you get to eat the healthy food you are choosing, plus you look like you've been more willing to invest time and effort into the friendship. You come out of this looking like the better person, that's all I'm saying...

There is also the perception that cooking - especially healthy cooking - takes so much time. This is another one of those lies we tell ourselves when what we really want to do is go out and grab dinner at our favourite place. Too much time? More time than getting ready to go out (most of us will at least do a cursory tidy up before leaving the house after a day at work or looking after the kids), getting in the car, driving through the traffic, waiting to be seated, waiting to order, waiting to be served, eating, waiting to see the inevitable desert menu because it feels rude to say no, eating the dessert you had no intention of having when you left the house but you're here now so you might as well, waiting to pay, getting back in the car, driving home (hopefully less traffic now) and flopping in front of the TV because you ended up eating more than you intended and now you're too full to do those jobs you wanted to get ticked off the list tonight? Often, depending on your personality type and how much you want or need to lose weight, then there will be the time required for a cycle of self-loathing to fit in there before bed as well.

The perception of time and convenience is a funny old thing, isn't it...

So I'm going to start from a 'can't cook, don't cook' perspective and anything you already do in your life that constitutes meal preparation is a bonus. Of course, I'm not saying I'm going to turn you into a great chef after reading a short book that isn't about cooking for the most part. But I will go through the relatively simple process of how to get there. The rest, my friend, is up to you to roll your sleeves up, dust off those appliances that sit unloved either on the work surface or in a cupboard somewhere, and begin.

The first simple step to getting there and staying there is this: lower your expectations.

The majority of books I've read, no matter which food alternative lifestyle they're representing, start with the promise of a healthy and tasty alternative that is so easy to do. Am I right? When was the last time you picked up a cook book and the introduction said that the recipes were going to be tricky, especially if you've never cooked before and have no idea what you're doing. Oh, and you'll probably only manage to make them just about edible for the first few times. How many say, *ignore the glossy bright picture on the opposite page, you'll never get it to look like that, even once you have done it enough times that now it actually tastes good?* Zero. It would be a terrible marketing approach for a cookbook to take.

Luckily, I'm not trying to sell you a cookbook, I'm trying to help you change your approach to food in a realistic and sustainable way. So start small. Lower your expectations.

This is especially true in those first few weeks of going sugar-free. This is the point at which you are going through withdrawal and your taste buds are changing. You will be having moments of cravings when nothing other than something really sweet seems worth it and, for a lot of people, moments when they suddenly seem to lose their appetite completely. That's enough of a shock on your body and mind without having to spend eight hours in the kitchen whipping up a three course meal.

The first thing you're going to master the art of creating: a large glass of water. You'll need a lot of water over the next few days. Don't worry about your body storing it. It will be too busy getting rid of it. Even though you won't necessarily be going ultra-low carb (although the lower you go, the more likely this is to happen), your body will begin to use its glycogen stores for some instant energy and jettison water as it goes. Plus, most people never drink enough anyway, so it's the easiest way to start. I set an alarm on my phone to quietly buzz in my pocket every hour as a reminder. When you're running around after kids or sitting in an office, it's easy to get engrossed and forget to do even this apparently simple step. Don't trust yourself to remember. Brains actually aren't very good at that, as you've probably noticed the last time you went to go shopping and walked out with half the things you'd intended to buy missing from your bag. So be realistic and set yourself up for success. Find some way of reminding yourself frequently enough throughout the day to have a drink.

Right, now onto the food itself.

Maybe when you went shopping, you put something in your basket that you've never tried before. If so, I commend you for being brave. Research a few recipes for it online and use that as a spark of enthusiasm to get you into the kitchen. If you only chose foods that you were familiar with, but still have never cooked before, you'll probably still need to do a bit of research to check cooking times and temperatures. Depending on your skill level, it's not my intention to make you go sugar-free for two weeks through a lack of choice due to food poisoning. Handle raw meat carefully and don't let it contaminate other foods via either your work surface or your hands. Wash fruit and vegetables before using (although let's be honest, who does that most of the time? Nevertheless, I've warned you that you should. All usual legal disclaimers apply).

There, I told you the basics were simple.

For weeks one and two, where food is going to taste strange and suddenly appear like an obstacle to the sweet stuff your body is telling you it needs, don't go fancy and don't feel like you've got to cook yourself a different dinner every night. You'll take a long time making food that won't taste like it's living up to what you expected and you'll begin to feel demoralised. At least by setting your standards low and consistent, you will be able to focus on getting through the withdrawal without the feeling of unsustainability, both in terms of time and your cooking ability.

I read somewhere long ago that those people who maintain consistently healthy bodies, whether they are pro athletes or just regular people, are the ones who treat food as fuel for breakfast and lunch. This makes utter sense to me. Your brain can only handle making so many decisions each day. That has been proven by science. The more decisions it needs to make, on anything, the more worn out it gets. Apparently, your brain will give the same amount of weight to making a decision about breakfast as it will to deciding whether or not to sign off a project with a million dollar budget. So the more decisions you make, the sooner its ability to do so effectively runs out. Ever notice that your decision making power is a little bit weaker by evening? Your brain seems to find it harder to make the right choice with enough clarity and determination to stick with it? This is known as decision fatigue and it has very real consequences. Few people go on ice cream binges mid morning, but by the evening, after a long and tiring day of living, there are very few people who haven't caved to this at some point. You can substitute ice cream for wine, beer, cake, chips, weakness of your choice, the principle still applies.

So eliminate options right from the start. Choose

your breakfast and stick with it. Choose your lunch and stick with it. Preferably pick ones that are as quick and simple as possible. They are your fuel meals.

If you've found a no added sugar, high fibre breakfast cereal that you're going to give a go, then sprinkle some seeds and berries and even if you don't enjoy the taste right now, begin to enjoy the consistency of starting your day off with success. You will also take advantage of waking up with that fresh batch of willpower and decision making ability and making it last longer. It all helps.

Lunch is easy too. Grilled chicken, salad - even take some low sugar bread out of your allowance and make a sandwich. Just make sure you don't add any dressings or mayonnaise. Certainly no low fat spread, made from goodness knows what. At times like this it is often tempting to think that you can carry on buying pre-packaged salads and sandwiches, if that is what you are already used to doing. Sadly, even though they can look innocent enough on the outside and no different to ones you could make yourself, most of them use added sugar to preserve any meat and give it a bit of flavour once it's been vacuum sealed for a month. Dressings that come with salad bowls can cover a multitude of sins as well and let's face it - when you have the packet there, it's just another bout of willpower to have to resist adding 'just a little bit to taste'. Then before you know it, you've added the whole lot and the slippery slope begins.

For these two meals, find what works and stick with it. Don't buy into the myth that you have to make lunch interesting, especially if you're one of those people who eat it at your desk while surfing the internet or working and will have no recollection of eating anyway.

If you love cooking (or if you learn to love cooking), then you might want to take the time to do it every evening. You might make it part of a social activity, or a chance to catch up with loved ones (how very quaint in today's world). That's a great place to be in. But if you don't have either the time or the inclination to be social and you actually haven't learned to enjoy it yet, then you need a Plan B.

The first is not to cook every evening. Like everything else in life, it's easier to be more productive when you batch things. If you can afford to be buying books, then I'm going to go out on a limb and assume you probably have a refrigerator and a freezer. Most likely a microwave too, but the oven is a perfectly acceptable way of reheating food if you have any moral objections to putting your food in the magic box. It is just as easy to make things for four meals as it is for two. Use that to your advantage.

Another simple yet annoying reality is the more you do something, the better you get at it. Chopping, peeling, knowing by sight and feel how long something is going to take to cook, they all get much easier the more you do them. Plus, frozen vegetables are an easy alternative in many cases, so all the chopping and peeling is done for you. They don't take any longer to cook and nutrient wise, you can often get more benefits than from an old carrot that has been sitting in some storeroom for a week in the dark waiting to come into stock rotation anyway. Grilled meat, fish and poultry can be cooked with a plate of vegetables in less than 15 minutes. It may not sound exotic, but if you have a time emergency, there is no excuse for grabbing a takeaway instead.

Does grilled chicken and vegetables sound boring to you? Throw on some herbs and spices and you've got a meal that spans global cuisine. A few dashes of five spice and suddenly you're eating Asian style. Some turmeric and cumin seeds and you're eating Indian.

Mediterranean herbs and you're going down the Italian route. It really is that simple and you just experiment until you find the flavour style and intensity that's right for you. Once you've kicked the sugar habit, you'll discover that the flavours become more intense anyway as a natural result of your palette changing over time.

As I said right at the beginning, this is a lifestyle change, so you have to *want* to do it. I'm just attempting to dismantle the myths around the impossible, whilst not lulling you into a false sense of security. You will still have to do things, make changes, and that is hard enough in itself. But cooking isn't an excuse to not to give it a go, even if your current level of expertise is making toast and you've never even turned your oven on.

CHAPTER SEVEN: FAST FOOD EMERGENCIES

So, you've bought the right food, taught yourself to love cooking, so it's all plain sailing from here right? Wrong. Why? Because life happens, that's why.

No matter how careful you are, no matter how much thought you put into it, things don't always go to plan. Those times when you get stuck during travel and waiting another four hours to eat at your final destination simply is not going to happen. Or when the food you'd planned to prepare smells slightly suspicious because you got it out of the refrigerator this morning to reach for something in the back and then somehow forgot to put it back.

Or, the most honest and likely scenario of all: you've had a bad day and the prospect of just about anything seems to require too much decision making and will power.

Those days are going to happen and as long as you don't use them as an excuse to eat fast food alternatives every day, then you don't have to derail everything for the occasional one. Knowledge is once again power, assuming you take it and use it in your favour.

Fast food joints, whatever they're selling as their main product, will mostly likely have at least one product that fits in with the sugar-free lifestyle. To save you arriving at your fast food emergency and spending fifteen minutes trying to get their website up on your phone so you can review the sugar content of every single one of their products, often including the ones that they no longer serve or offer somewhere else around the globe (yes, I've done that, far too many times) start from this point: chicken.

If you are vegetarian or vegan, you've probably spent longer than I have already hunting down the poor showings at any food establishment outside a big city, so you're going to be more adept than I am at this anyway. For the purposes of this section, I'm going to assume that you're a meat eater.

So, chicken. Fried chicken, at less than 0.5g of sugar per piece at the most well known establishment, is totally allowed on the sugar-free diet. Plus, because we don't care about fat and calories anymore because our bodies at this point register food correctly and tell us when we are full, we don't have to worry about eating the skin and tasty bits. There is a simple joy in letting go of decades of advice to cut off the skin because that is where the fat is. Don't get me wrong, I still choose to eat chicken without skin most of the time, but not worrying about it is certainly liberating.

Assuming you're at a fast food joint that sells burgers more than chicken, then you've still got the chicken option. Even the most famous place of all has chicken nuggets. As long as you avoid the dips (be prepared for them to look at you like you've just confessed to killing kittens when you reply 'none, thank you' in response to the server asking which ones you would like), then you can eat them without worry or care.

The bad news... commercial pizza is not allowed. The sauce is integral to the product and let's face it, you wouldn't want a pizza without it. But at between 5-8g per slice for most options (the highest one I found before I had to stop looking because it was making me sad, was 12g per slice), this is simply too high. Plus, don't fool yourself that you'll just have one slice. That never happens. If you've mastered the love of cooking to the point where you want to give it a go, then have your pizza fix at home. There are low sugar recipes available online and whilst not perfect, at least you'll be able to control what goes in them.

Mexican food has long been a roadside staple in America and that delicious trend is spreading around many parts of the world. Here, the problem is that independent stalls can show significant variation, making it hard to pick a guaranteed good option. Throw on the possibility of commercial bought extras and you're certain to be bumping up the sugar as a preservative. The quality of the outlet will make a huge difference; if you're paying rock bottom prices for a quick fill up then you know the ingredients will be cheap and easy to use to compensate for the potential profit loss. If you find yourself with Mexican food as your only option, then stick with something that is more meat than sauce and corn rather than flour tortillas or tacos. Then just enjoy it. It's an emergency, remember, so it's not going to happen again anytime soon anyway is it? That was in my stern voice by the way, just in case you were reading it and actively planning in cheat days. Say it with me. *Emergencies only.*

Fish n chips - this one is clearly aimed at fellow British and Antipodean readers more than American ones - are okay in a pinch. Just don't use it as an excuse to go mad and have the giant special with all the sauces and extras. Just a small fish and chips is high carb and high fat, but the sugar element, from every nutritional piece of information I've been able to track down, indicates it is low. As there are very few chain style fish and chip shops, this makes controlling the consistency very hard, but if you want to be doubly sure, then take off the batter and just eat the fish inside. An increasing number of restaurants are now even offering grilled options if you ask. Regular chips - I say regular because you can get all kinds of tasty coatings that throw the rule book out - are just potatoes in lots of oil, and at less than 1% sugar, they are allowed on the sugar-free way of living even if they're just a beautiful distant memory on super low carb.

Sushi has been often sold as a healthy and tasty alternative to the big name western fast food restaurants. Sadly, the thing that makes the rice stick together so well is sugar. So no matter what tasty and healthy low sugar option is wrapped up like a little present inside, the whole thing is encased in a layer of sweetness. Again, it's hard to pin down the exact nutritional values as a product like this can vary wildly, but you're looking at about 10g per sushi roll. Which, delicious as it may be, probably isn't going to be satisfying enough to stop you having a second. On a broader takeaway scale, Chinese, Thai, Cantonese, Malaysian etc are generally completely off limits. The sauces in commercial versions of these foods (and if you're in a high end restaurant, it's not exactly a fast food emergency, is it?) are all very high in sugar which explains why you can eat a giant portion until you are utterly stuffed, yet somehow feel curiously empty just a few hours later.

Finally, if you are frequently on the road, then a good quality protein bar can be an occasional solution. This needs some pre-thought and preparation, but it can save you from completely derailing yourself in an emergency. Not all protein bars are created equal, so it is best to shop around. With the main emphasis being – obviously – on the protein content, it is easy to overlook the other nasties that may be in there. However, there are some better options, such as Quest bars, that are aimed at also being low carb and low sugar. I always thought they were hugely expensive for a snack bar, but once your appetite system has reset, then they really can work as a meal replacement. Looking at them as half the price of a standard lunch makes it a more sensible option in many cases. You simply have to make sure that you take the time up front to purchase the ones that are right for you and then make sure they will be there when you need them, in your bag or in the car.

So, with emergency situations out of the way, you should be well on the way to living the sugar-free lifestyle. But if you're reading this all the way through before starting (which I'm going to assume that, as a normal person, you probably are), then you'll probably still be thinking about weight loss, rather than overall health. Are you gearing up to feel the burn...?

CHAPTER EIGHT: EXERCISE

There is a tendency when beginning any new diet to also begin a (generally short-lived) intense exercise regime. Again, that is because most people make these food choices to lose weight, rather than to live a healthier lifestyle. The double hit of reduced calories and an expensive new gym wardrobe or piece of wonder equipment is surely the best way to do it, right?

I would say, from my own experience, no. Not for this. The changes to your body that come through eliminating sugar from your diet are hard enough to deal with on their own, so throwing a sudden gruelling exercise regime into the mix and you're going to be in a world of pain.

Interestingly, there have been recent discoveries around a gene that makes some people resistant to exercise when it comes to burning enough fat to lose weight. An interesting thought. The numbers are apparently around 30% of the population, although my money is on 95% of readers thinking it might be them.

Why? Because the body is a very, very efficient machine. It is designed to work optimally without actually expending much energy (therefore burning few calories).

For years, in my quest to maintain a healthy weight easily, I still never got into going to the gym. The maths never held up for me that exercise was the best way to lose weight. For the average person - again, I'm excluding athletes and the super fit here - going flat out at the gym for an hour can burn off a decent burger. Not the rest of the meal, but the burger. If you approach the session in a more relaxed manner, then you might not even manage to burn off that. You're a lean mean fighting machine naturally, designed to stay alive for a long time and keep on the move, even when the food supply is irregular. Your body doesn't *want* to burn calories this way. The best way of maintaining a healthy constant is to work on getting your body used to eating the food it is meant to eat *first*.

Now, before you take it that I am advocating a complete couch surfing lifestyle, I'm not. Moderate exercise is good for all of us. It builds and maintains muscle mass and contributes to keeping our heart and lungs healthy. It has been proven to create hormones to boost mental health too. Exercise is very important. I just don't believe it's the *key* to losing weight on a diet. Again, this is about a healthy way of living, but it is another of those myths that goes hand-in-hand with what brought you here, so it needs to be addressed.

So what should you do? Let's assume for now that you're a complete exercise novice. On a good day, you congratulate yourself for taking the stairs rather than any kind of mechanical alternative. So start with a twenty minute walk. As brisk as you can physically manage.

That's it.

Get your body used to moving again and begin to build another habit alongside your new food habits.

This is the easiest thing to do because it doesn't require any investment from you other than time. You can spare twenty minutes to do this. You don't need any fancy clothes and you don't need any expensive equipment. If you're crippled by social anxiety, you don't even need to leave the house. If you live across two or more floors, even better. Throw in climbing the stairs a few times and you've gone extra hard. The key is just to start walking and not stop for twenty minutes.

I can understand the appeal in going at top speed straight out the gate. We live in a world of instant gratification and we want to see instant results. Hitting on all fronts therefore seems like the most logical approach. Yet the majority of people make the same New Year's resolution around ten times before doing anything that sticks. Often that resolution is around losing weight and getting fit. It's almost a cliché that the gym is always too busy to move in January yet virtually empty by February. People start with good intentions and they try to change everything at once. We are, at heart, creatures of habit. Think back to chapter four. You're not going to become a different person overnight and somehow sustain it with willpower alone. Be kind to yourself. Start with eliminating added sugar from your diet, give your body time to adjust to a new way of living and you'll probably find you want to move it more anyway. Losing weight will happen naturally and you won't have to worry about finding the motivation to get to the gym. After a few days, or a week, increase to thirty minutes. If setting aside a single block of time like thirty minutes is too long, then steal two blocks of twenty minutes from your day. You can then increase to the level you want. If you decide that this whole exercise thing is for you after all, you can try jogging. Or swimming. Or you can join a gym and go all out. I've got some dumbbells at home that I hold whilst walking to strengthen my core and build a little bit of extra muscle mass. I probably look like a complete idiot to anyone who is walking by and happens to glance through the window, but I don't really care. I haven't had to waste time putting on exercise clothes, sitting in traffic to get to the gym, exercise and then do the same in reverse to get my workout, effectively losing at least an hour of my day in order to get that twenty minutes of exercise in.

So, start small, build to being as vigorous as you can and want to be. Don't shun movement altogether. But don't set yourself up for pain and injury when your body is in the process of changing itself. Give it a chance to adjust. We're not doing the *lose ten pounds in three weeks for summer!* magazine diet here. Build a lifestyle where you can be at your desired health goals each day, not just for a week once every bikini season.

CHAPTER NINE: NOW GO DO IT

What next?

Hopefully, this little book has given you enough of the detail you need to be convinced - if you weren't already - to give the sugar-free lifestyle a chance. Most importantly, I hope that I haven't painted too demoralising a picture, but instead one that means you won't lapse straight away purely due to the shock of unexpected addiction and body changes.

Now, quite simply, it is time to give it a go.

The simple checklist of steps below has been condensed to give every realist trying to live sugar-free a quick and easy guide to work through. Rather than re-reading all of the chapters (although feel free to do so if you wish), just work through each phase and know that if you relapse, you can just pick up again at the step most relevant to you.

I've also included space here to document your own journey, so you can set yourself up for success.

Step One

Pick a day to begin, the sooner the better. Have a big birthday celebration this weekend? Don't try it before then. Chances are that you'll have some kind of food event each week, so there will never be a perfect time. That's okay. Unless it's a reason you absolutely can't get out of eating the food provided, then start by just picking a date. *Soon.* If that's today or tomorrow, then good for you, but you'll need to get through the next few steps now as well. Most importantly, write down the reasons why you want to be sugar-free.

My sugar-free start date:

_____

_____

Events in the next 30 days:

_____

_____

_____

_____

_____

_____

Why I want to be sugar-free:

_____

_____

_____

_____

_____

_____

_____

_____

_____

_____

_____

_____

_____

_____

_____

_____

_____

_____

Step Two

Get a habit tracker. I don't care whether you use paper or digital, you just have to be able to track your sugar-free days. Any other small habits can be captured here as well, like walking or drinking water frequently. I've included examples below, but there are more ideas in the *Resources* section at the end of the book.

Basic Habit Tracker Example

Day	Sugar Free	Water	Exercise
1	✖	✖	✖
2	✖	✖	✖
3	✖	✖	
4	✖	✖	
5		✖	✖
6	✖		
7	✖	✖	✖
8	✖	✖	✖
9	✖		
10	✖		
11			
12			
13			
14			

My Habit Tracker

Day			
1			
2			
3			
4			
5			
6			
7			
8			
9			
10			
11			
12			
13			
14			
15			

My Habit Tracker

Day			
16			
17			
18			
19			
20			
21			
22			
23			
24			
25			
26			
27			
28			
29			
30			
31			

Step Three

Take a good, long, honest look at your eating habits. Think about your weak times of day, or days of week. Look at the calendar. What do you need to be prepared for? There is no shame or blame going on here, just an honest moment with yourself so you can set yourself up to succeed, not to fail. Remember, you are going to be quitting an addictive behaviour. If you've ever done that before, then what are the ways you did it and the lessons you learned in the process? These will help guide you in the right direction towards the best way to remove sugar from your life that is right for you.

My bad sugar habits:

_____

_____

_____

_____

_____

_____

_____

My bad sugar habits:

_____

_____

_____

_____

_____

_____

_____

_____

_____

_____

_____

_____

Times of least willpower:

_____

_____

_____

_____

_____

_____

_____

_____

_____

_____

_____

_____

_____

_____

_____

Step Four

Get prepared to eat food that doesn't contain added sugar. If your house is full of chocolate, then you're going to struggle with temptation. Similarly, if you're a savoury person and there are sauces and dressings filling your cupboard and refrigerator, get rid of them. It feels very wrong throwing away perfectly good food, so if you can, give it to family or friends. They probably think you're mad for trying to do this anyway (they'll start to get more interested in a couple of months time when they see the change), but they'll usually take free food. By doing this, not only are you removing temptation, but also making the psychological commitment to do this for more than a few days, because you don't want to have to buy everything a second time when you already had perfectly good supplies of it before. Unless you're rolling in cash and completely restocking your kitchen is no big deal, then this is a great way of testing right now how committed you are to the plan.

Once you've got rid of the food you don't need, you'll need to replace it with the food that you want. Don't forget to grab those herbs and spices along the way.

How did that feel? Am I prepared?

_____

_____

_____

_____

_____

_____

_____

_____

_____

_____

_____

_____

_____

Step Five

Plan your food for that first week. Not much time to cook? Then set aside the time to do batch foods. Don't plan a gourmet week. Stick with the basics, make sure you know what you're having and that includes snack times.

There will be eating habits to break and if you are used to giving yourself a snack mid-afternoon every workday, when that sugar slump used to kick in (you know the one, where lunch is a distant memory but the clock says you've still got another two hours before you can leave work), then you'll need to replace your unhealthy snack with another one, at least in the short term.

Don't leave yourself vulnerable to your addiction and your habits. Certainly don't trust yourself to do the right thing on the day. Use the following pages to really think about how and what you intend to eat during this first week.

Monday

Breakfast:

_____

_____

_____

Lunch:

_____

_____

_____

Dinner:

_____

_____

_____

Snacks:

_____

_____

_____

Tuesday

Breakfast:

_____

_____

_____

Lunch:

_____

_____

_____

Dinner:

_____

_____

_____

Snacks:

_____

_____

_____

Wednesday

Breakfast:

_____

_____

_____

Lunch:

_____

_____

_____

Dinner:

_____

_____

_____

Snacks:

_____

_____

_____

Thursday

Breakfast:

_____

_____

_____

Lunch:

_____

_____

_____

Dinner:

_____

_____

_____

Snacks:

_____

_____

_____

Friday

Breakfast:

_____

_____

_____

Lunch:

_____

_____

_____

Dinner:

_____

_____

_____

Snacks:

_____

_____

_____

Saturday

Breakfast:

_____

_____

_____

Lunch:

_____

_____

_____

Dinner:

_____

_____

_____

Snacks:

_____

_____

_____

Sunday

Breakfast:

_____

_____

_____

Lunch:

_____

_____

_____

Dinner:

_____

_____

_____

Snacks:

_____

_____

_____

Step Six

The Big Day. Begin with a feeling of positivity and commitment. Keep that feeling going for as long as you can, it's a nice experience. The road ahead is going to get bumpy at times, so the more you can hold onto that feeling the better. Know your plan and stick with it. If you can, give yourself a twenty minute walk - outside if possible, but it's okay if not - and give yourself a big pat on the back at the end of the day. Mark the day off in your habit tracker for the food and the walk.

Congratulations. You have begun.

Step Seven

Get through the first week. I can't put it any clearer than that. Day one won't have felt too bad. Your body can handle the short term change and removing sugar doesn't mean a restriction in portion size or calories, so you won't be left feeling like you've tortured yourself. The next week will be reducing sugar from your diet or eliminating it completely. It will be tough. Start each day with commitment and allow yourself to enjoy the sense of achievement when you check off the day in your habit tracker at the end. Don't worry about responding to your feelings of hunger as they change; remember, you might not feel hungry at traditional meal times for a while and that's okay too. Eat when you need to, not when the clock tells you to.

Just keep going. You can do this, even when it feels like you can't.

Step Eight

The home stretch. This is the first month. Whether you go cold turkey or allow yourself to gradually remove sugar from your diet, you should be sugar-free by the end of the first month. If you allow the gentle removal to go much longer than that, you'll never actually get rid of it. You'll cling onto that comfort blanket just a little too long and then it will always be there. *One whole month.* Keep tracking your habits, give yourself props for any exercise and track that too. If you have a day where you slip up and break the habit streak, then pick yourself up, dust yourself off and begin again. Your goal is to get a full consistent month of sugar-free living. Keep going until you achieve that.

Step Nine

Take the time to enjoy your new life. Don't stop the habit tracker; it's a simple thing but it will give you much more success than willpower alone. Remember, your brain is designed to let you down and make the easiest choice, not the best one, when you are tired. External enforcement is a better way. Enjoy food tasting the way it should, enjoy your body feeling fitter, healthier and leaner. Enjoy people remarking on how good you look and asking if something has changed.

Don't let a bad day derail you.

And remember: if you fall off the wagon completely, that doesn't mean you can't ever climb back on. This time you'll be more prepared and will have learned the lesson of what made you fall off so you can see it coming next time. The whole experience of going sugar-free gets a little bit easier each time you restart.

Have faith in yourself. You can do this. I wish you every success and when the going gets tough, just keep going.

GET IN TOUCH

The decision to write this book came out of a burning passion to help people understand why they were struggling to lose and maintain weight, despite restricting their calories, exercising and generally making food something to be miserable about.

Those of my friends who saw the benefits, who even went through long periods of success, still had epic falls off the wagon, generally involving cake. Not me. I fell off the wagon for ice cream and holidays. But fall off the wagon I did.

I simply wanted to make it easier for other people to spot the pitfalls coming, so they could hold on tighter and achieve greater success, as well as becoming healthier individuals along the way.

If you have any experiences you'd like to share, then please get in touch at realist@sherrinicholds.com. I think the need for sugar awareness is going to continue to grow, so if I update this book, I'm happy to move from a sample size of one, to many, many more.

Similarly, if you're one of those scientist types who actually *really* understand this at a deep biochemical level and want to inform me of any errors, updates or alternative insights, then I'd love to hear from you too.

REFERENCES AND RESOURCES

For a free weekly meal planning guide and quick reference shopping list, head over to http://sherrinicholds.com/realist

Other useful websites

Increasingly, there are websites devoted to helping you remove the added sugar from your life. Realising you are not alone can go a long way towards keeping you on track. Two of the best places to start are:

David Gillespie http://www.howmuchsugar.com

Sarah Wilson https://iquitsugar.com

Habit trackers

As far as I am concerned, building sugar-free habits are the best way to help you quit sugar and then stay off it for good. There are many great ones out there and if you want to go the digital route, then I would suggest choosing one that suits your style. It needs to appeal to you emotionally as well as visually, or you won't become invested in using it. I use https://www.coach.me and have done for several years, so I can personally recommend this one. Others include:

http://www.stridesapp.com

http://productiveapp.io

http://balancedapp.com

http://streaksapp.com

Not everyone will see the appeal in a digital app. For those of you who like to go analogue and keep track of things with good old-fashioned pen and paper, then I can also recommend heading over to http://bulletjournal.com and taking a look at that system. Many users in the Bullet Journal community have modified the system with habit and health tracking in mind, so it is a great place to start.

Articles and further information

If you're looking for more information to support the theory in this book and find out more about the research that made me take giving up sugar seriously, then there are plenty of articles online. For those of your so inclined, there are plenty of additional research articles published in journals requiring a fee. Because there is a cost associated with membership, I have tried to avoid highlighting them here. However, below are just a handful of the places you can go to begin.

http://www.jci.org/articles/view/37385#sd

http://www.degruyter.com/view/j/hmbci.2015.22.is sue-2/hmbci-2015-0009/hmbci-2015-0009.xml

https://publichealthmatters.blog.gov.uk/2015/07/1 7/expert-interview-new-sugar-recommendations/

http://www.who.int/mediacentre/news/releases/20 15/sugar-guideline/en/

Finally...

LEGO® is a trademark of the LEGO Group of companies which does not sponsor, authorize or endorse this book.

Quest Bar is a trademark of Quest Nutrition LLC which does not sponsor, authorize or endorse this book.

ACKNOWLEDGEMENTS

Quite simply, this book is for my friends, who inspire me daily with their pragmatic yet humorous approaches to all of life's challenges, not just diet and lifestyle. I'd also like to thank my Dreamers writing group, who for the past few years have been a constant source of encouragement and support. Catherine, especially, provided some invaluable insights during the editing of this book. I wouldn't have been able to write this book without the scientists and nutritionists who are challenging the status quo and making the facts accessible to us regular people. Last, but by no means least, a huge thank you to Anna, who has been a sounding board for this book for nearly a year. Without your constant cheer-leading and sacrifices, I simply wouldn't be able to do this thing I love.

ABOUT THE AUTHOR

Sherri Nicholds is an independent author and freelancer. A productivity and efficiency geek, she has spent years making it her mission to study, systematize and improve every area of her life. This in turn led to her becoming a passionate advocate of sugar-free living. She now spends much of her time sharing the tips and tricks she has learnt along the way with others.

Along with writing and personal development, she is a keen traveler and is always in search of the next adventure.

Printed in Great Britain
by Amazon

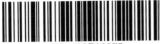